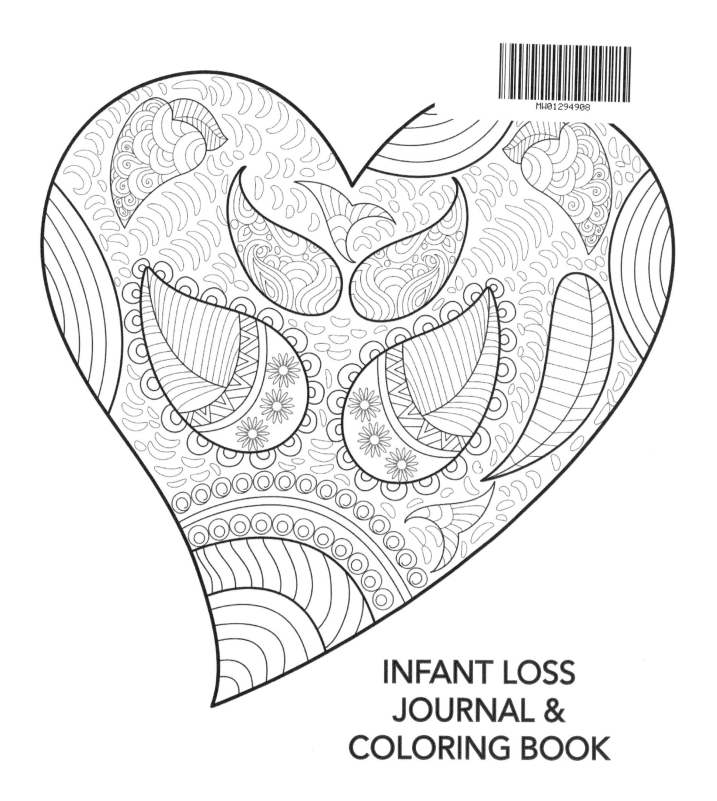

INFANT LOSS JOURNAL & COLORING BOOK

Copyright © 2019 Christina Moyer
ISBN: 9781691058969
All rights reserved.
No part of this book may be reproduced or redistributed without express permission from the author and publishing company. Licensed graphics used with all appropriate commercial licenses.

My Story...

My daughter, Mia Jenifer Moyer was born March 4, 2002. Oh, I miss her. I think of her often. I wonder what she would be doing now or what she would look like.

Thinking back, I wonder how I made it through. I hope you find comfort by reading my story and using the journaling and coloring pages in your healing.

"Blessed are they that mourn: for they shall be comforted"- Matthew 5:4

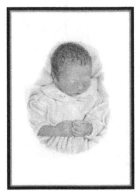

Mia was our second born. I was surprised when I got pregnant as we weren't trying at the time. Our first daughter just turned 2 when I found out I was pregnant.

She was so excited to have a baby brother or sister. We didn't want to find out what we were having until she/he was born.

I was having a smooth pregnancy until around 32 weeks. The doctor said I was measuring small. They did an ultrasound and found nothing wrong.

Then one day when I was 34 weeks, I felt pain. It felt like labor pain. I called the doctor and she thought maybe I ate something bad that day. I told her I didn't. She said to come to the hospital right away.

So I called my husband at work and he rushed home. We headed to the hospital. I was in so much pain. The doctor was at the front desk and they immediately took me to a room. I was told later that the doctor said I was as "white as a ghost".

When we were in the room, the nurse put a tight monitor around my belly. She kept trying to find the heartbeat. I could tell she was making excuses for not finding it.

Then the doctor came in. She looked on the ultrasound machine and I could tell she couldn't find the heartbeat either. I kept praying for some miracle.

But it didn't happen. The doctor turned and looked at my husband and I and said, "I'm sorry, I can't find a heartbeat"

The next few hours were a blur to me. I delivered Mia naturally as my body was already going into labor. That is why I was experiencing so much pain.

The hospital was so wonderful. They let us hold her for as long as we wanted. My Mom, Sister and My Husband's Parents all came to see us. The nurse's dressed her in their preemie outfits that they had and took many pictures of her.

After a few hours, we realized we needed to say goodbye. It was so hard for me to say goodbye to my baby.

We spent the night in the hospital. I kept waking up thinking about all that had happened. Nurses were coming in and checking up on me all the time. The doctor released me the next day.

We went home in a state of shock. **What had just happened?** How could I lose my baby? Everything was fine until yesterday.

I often heard the hardest thing for someone to do is bury a child. I totally agree.

I didn't realize it until afterwards, but my husband had a hard time making the funeral arrangements. He tried to call the funeral home twice and just couldn't. He said he stared at the phone thinking, "Do I really have to do this?"

The funeral home and cemetery were wonderful as they provided their services including the burial plot and funeral services at no charge. We did have to pay for a coffin, which came in two sizes. That was very hard for us to pick out a coffin for our daughter. She is in Babyland with all the other babies.

We decided to have a private viewing at the funeral home with just immediate family. We invited a few people to the funeral service at the grave site. Word got out and we were so amazed as about 50 people come to the funeral. We were so blessed to have our family and friends there for support.

"Mommy, why are you crying?"

That is what my 2 1/2 year old said to me every day. Even though she didn't understand, she knew I was sad. She wanted to help me and she did tremendously.

She helped me get up out of bed every day. She would give me hugs and kisses and tell me it is okay. She kept telling me she loved me.

Now, she is an adult and we share that bond. We talk about Mia a lot and she tells everyone she has a sister that died. She tells them she is in Heaven with Jesus.

On Mia's first birthday, we had a birthday celebration for her. Alison blew out Mia's candles and my husband said, "Happy Birthday Mia". Alison said, "She is having the best birthday ever!" We both said, "Yes, she is".

Jesus said, "Let the little children come to me." - Mark 10:14

May you find comfort in my story, this journal and coloring book and know you are not alone.

Christina

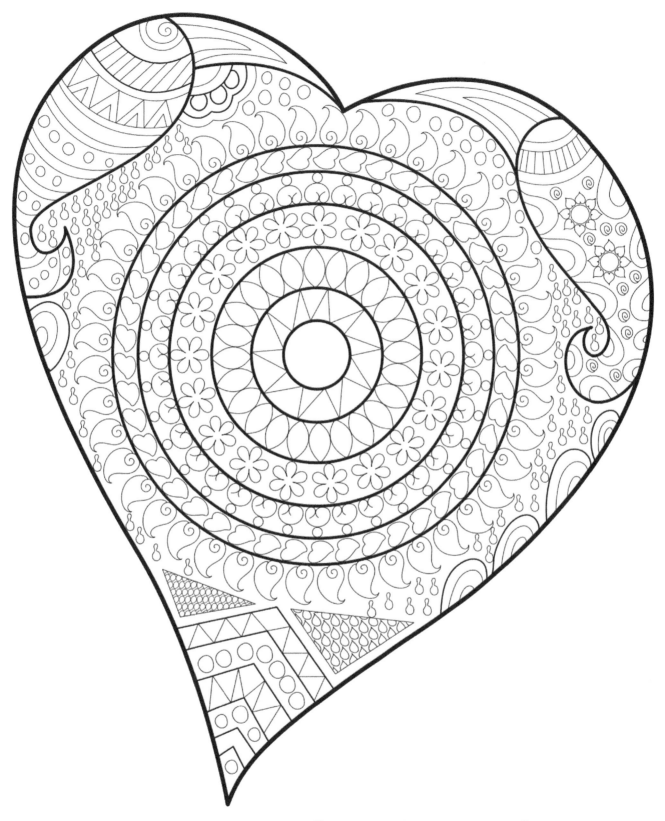

Blessed are those who mourn, for they will be comforted. - Matthew 6:4

When I first found out I was pregnant...

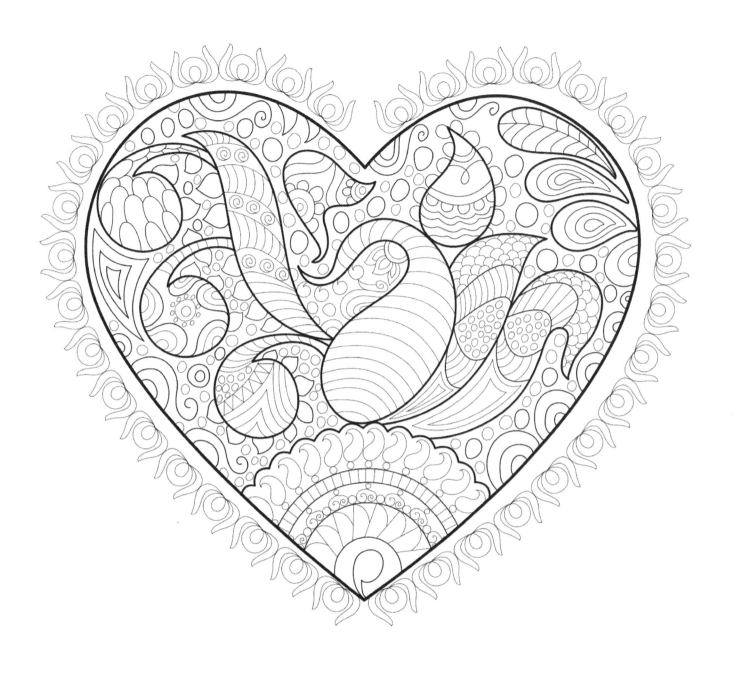

God is the strength of my heart and my portion forever.
Psalm 73:26

What my dreams were for this baby...

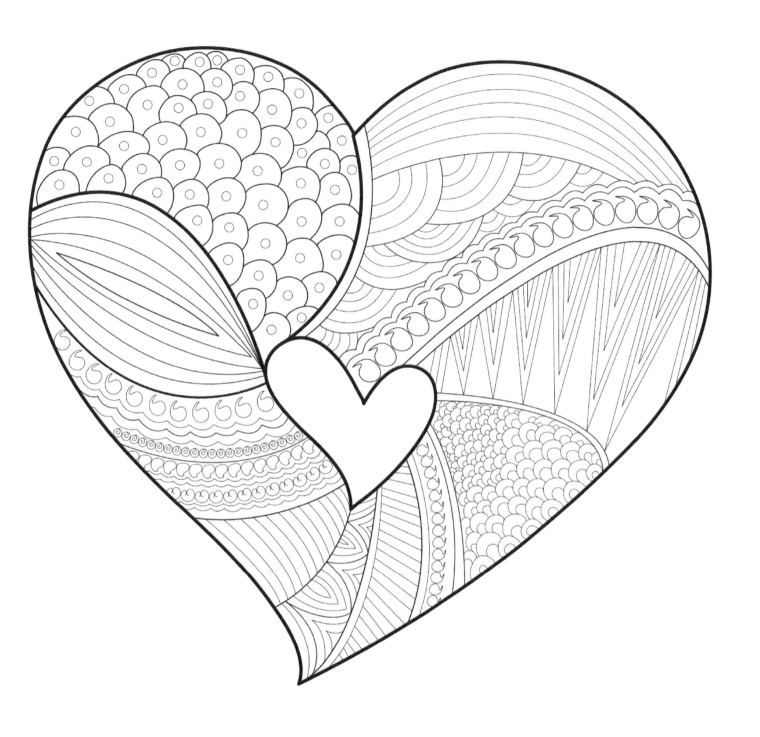

"Before I formed you in the womb I knew you"
Jeremiah 1:5

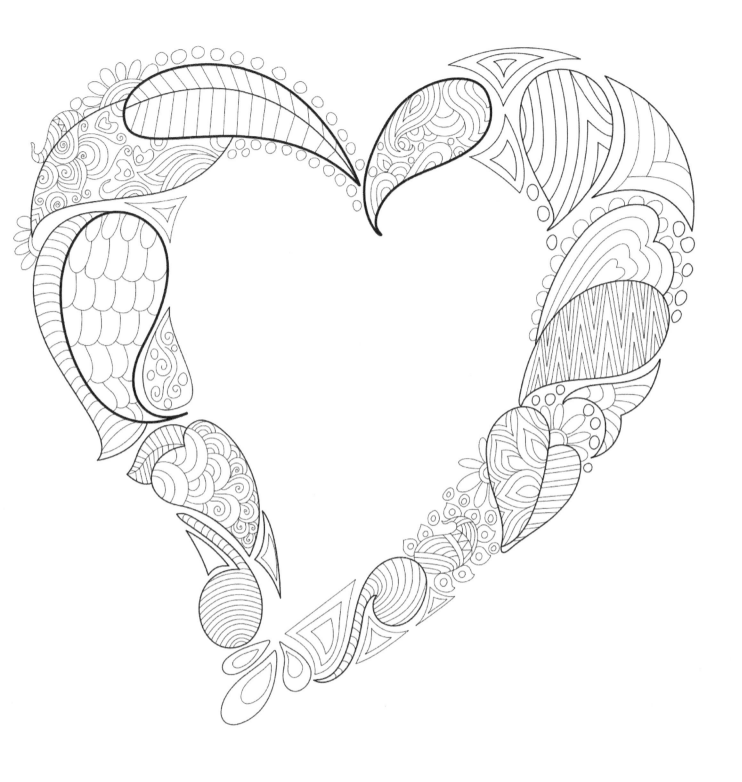

Sharing my story even if it was in a private journal, was a comfort to me in my healing. I encourage you to share your story on the next pages.

My Story...

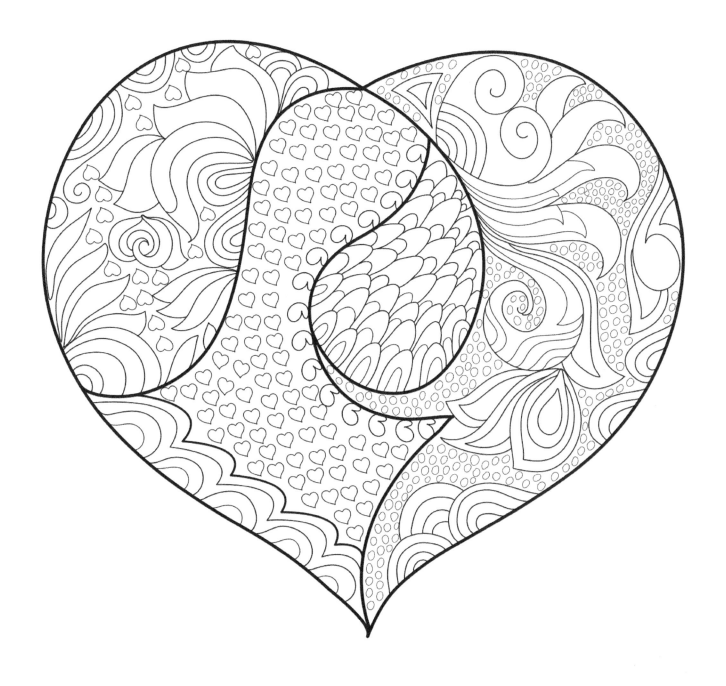

Music was a big help in my healing.
"Blessed Be Your Name" was a big comfort to me.

I encourage you to find a song that is an encouragement to you.

How Do I Feel Today?

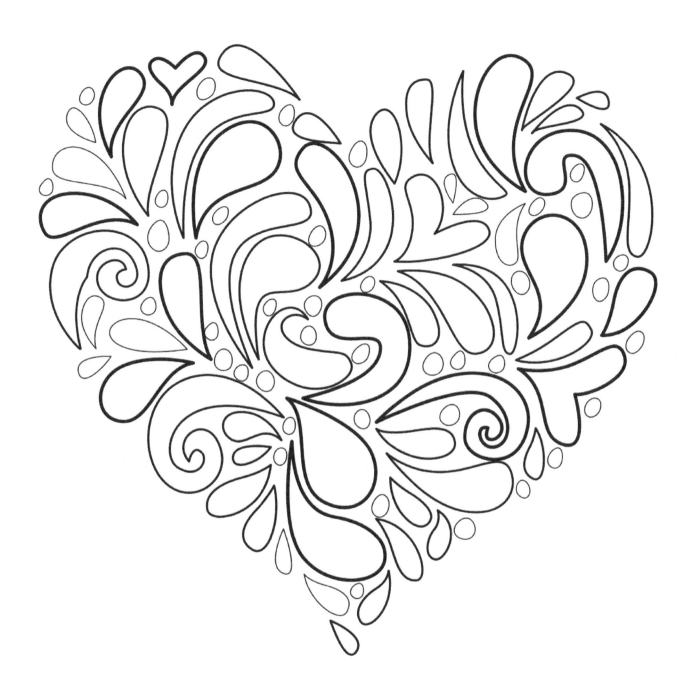

Letting others help me was a benefit in my healing. Just someone there to listen or be there even when I didn't want to talk was such an encouragement.

How Do I Feel Today?

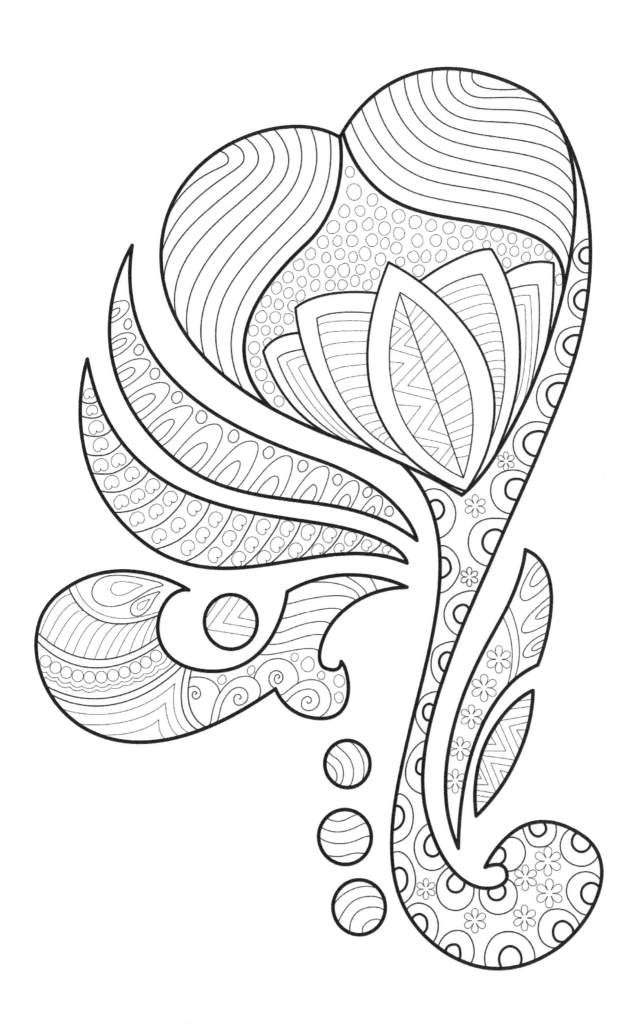

How Do I Feel Today?

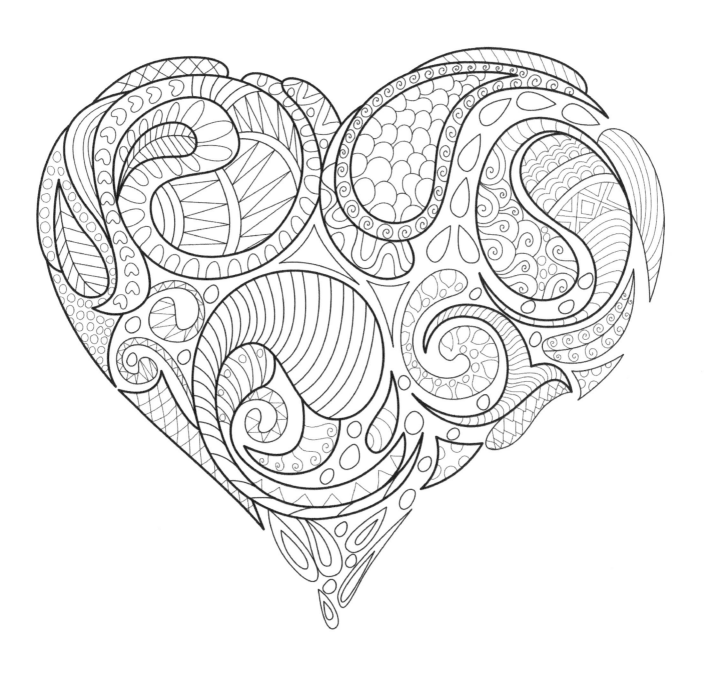

Painting and creating was a help in my healing. Taking pictures of God's creation and going to a painting class was a way for me to express my feelings.

How Do I Feel Today?

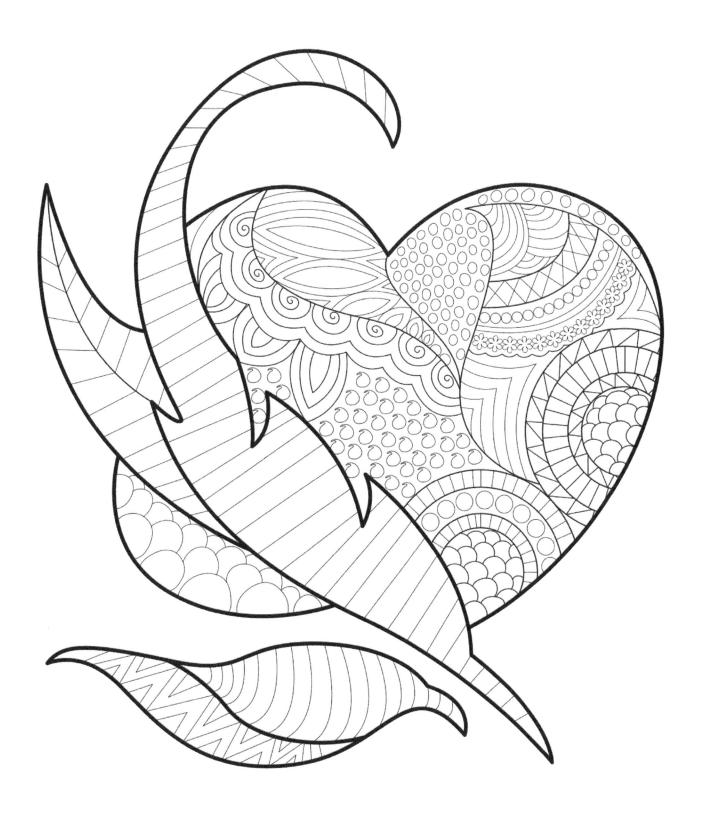

How Do I Feel Today?

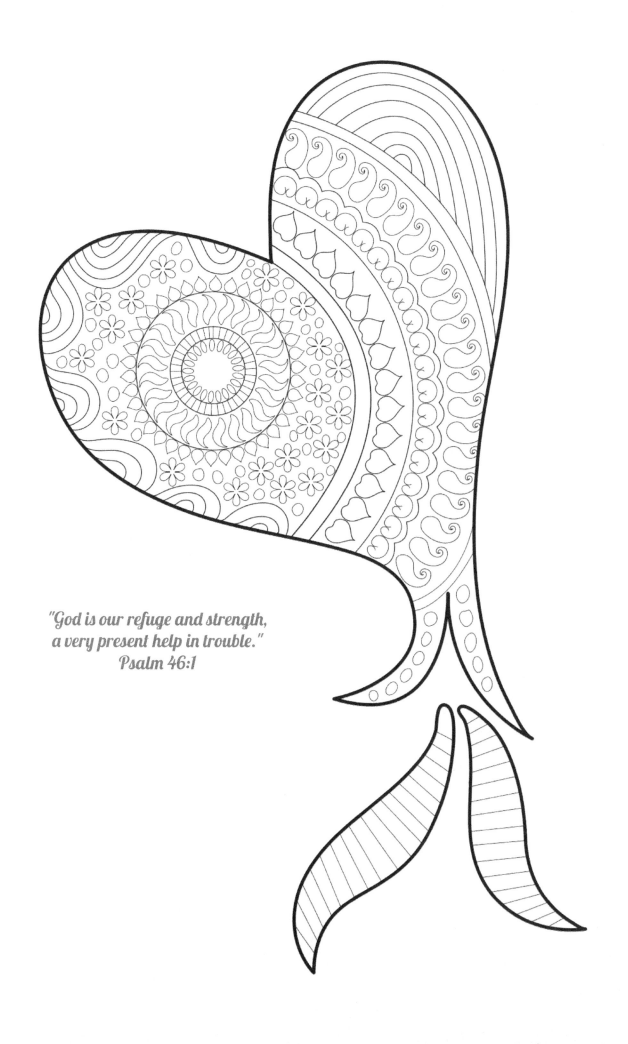

"God is our refuge and strength,
a very present help in trouble."
Psalm 46:1

How Do I Feel Today?

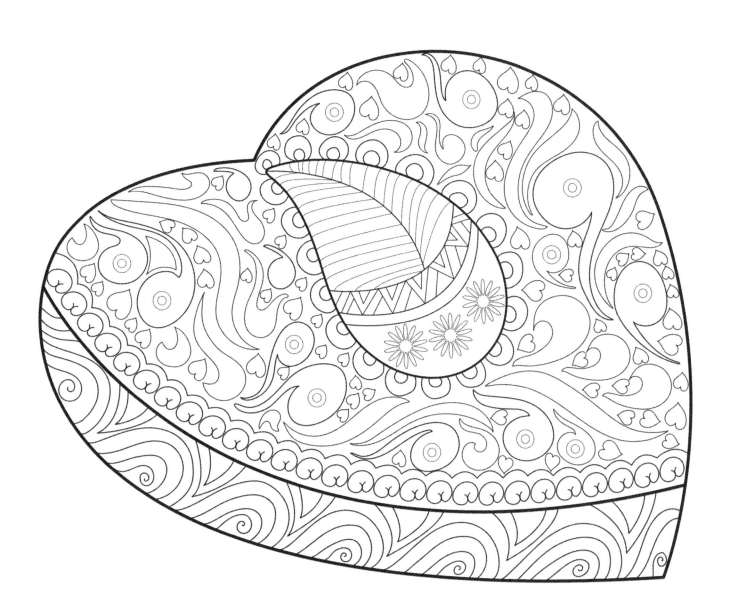

How Do I Feel Today?

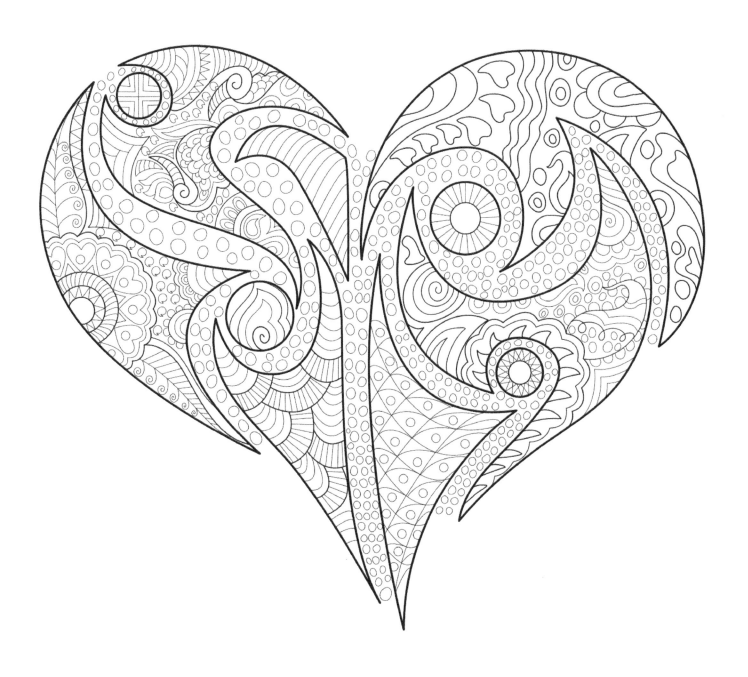

The Lord is near to the brokenhearted, and saves the crushed in spirit.
Psalm 34:18

How Do I Feel Today?

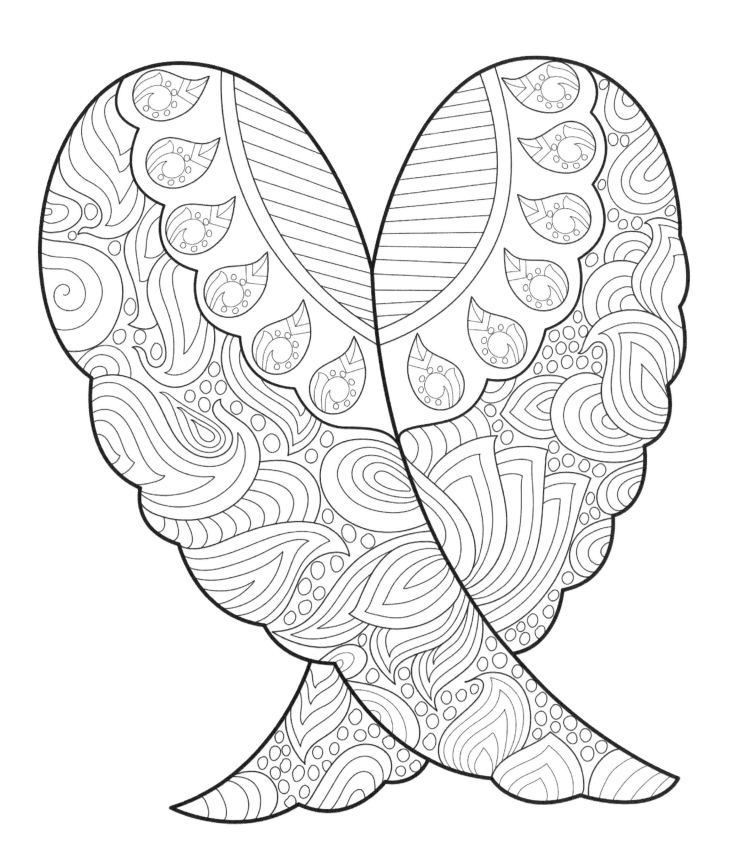

How Do I Feel Today?

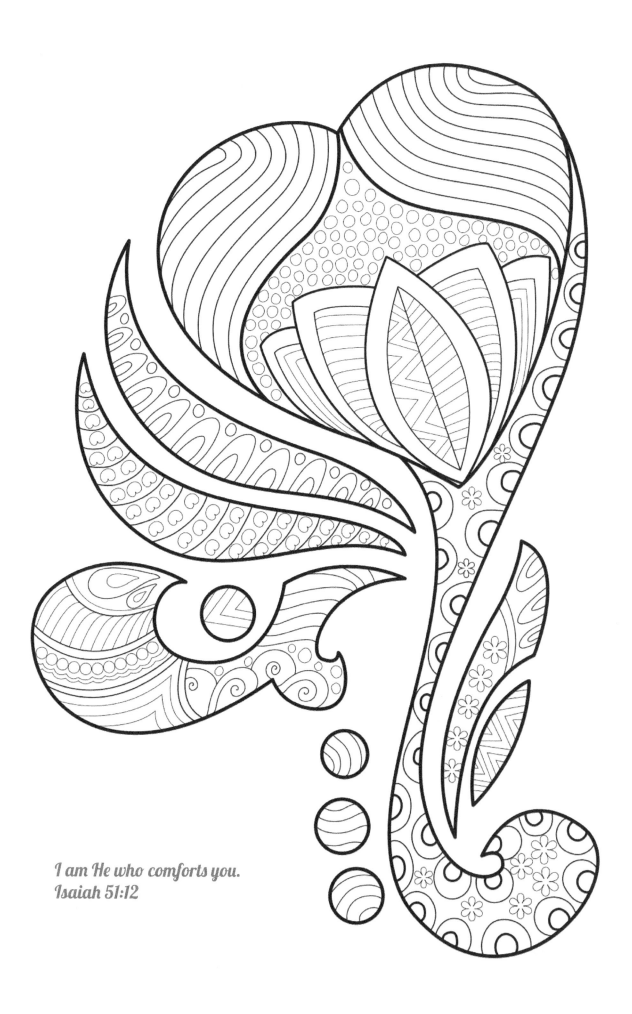

I am He who comforts you.
Isaiah 51:12

How Do I Feel Today?

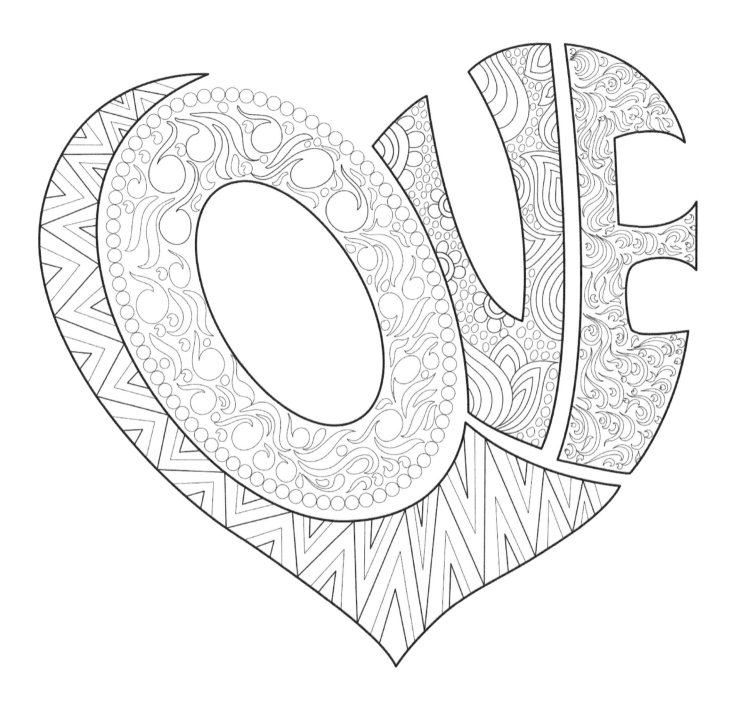

Thanks for going through this journey. I hope my story and these pages helped you to start to heal. It is a long process and won't go away quickly but as each day passes it does get better.

Know, you are loved.

Made in the USA
Middletown, DE
06 June 2023